Introduction

Usually there is a lot of confusion over the term Veganism. Let's look at what it really means:

Veganism is a philosophy, diet, and a lifestyle. Vegans survive on only products from the Plant Kingdom. They recognize the rights and value of all living creatures and follow the Golden Rule.

Not only do Vegans value the life of all living creatures, but they also show compassion, kindness, and justice to everything and everyone as well.

This is one of the main reason why you don't see Vegans at zoos nor aquariums. They do not support animal exploitations in any form. For someone to follow truly follow veganism, they will have an arduous but self-fulfilling journey ahead of them.

To clarify:

Vegetarianism is basically a lifestyle in which people consume animal related products like milk, yogurt, butter, eggs, etc. But they refrain only from consuming meat and meat products.

Veganism on the other hand, is a lifestyle where people lack the consumption of meat and animal related products in their everyday diet; this includes milk, butter, eggs, etc.

In addition, Vegans refrain from consumption or involvement with ANY and ALL animal products.

From clothing to adornments, it is hard to believe that we are surrounded by a great deal of animal related products. Fortunately, there are plenty of affordable and accessible alternatives to just about everything.

A Vegan diet is a diet where an individual tries to exclude any and all form of produce and edible product that comes from animals such as meat.

This also includes other products that come from animals such as milk or eggs. To its followers, going vegan means more than just following a diet, it is a lifestyle. Many support the Vegan diet in hopes of abolishing animal cruelty and exploitation from the planet.

Now keep in mind, there is a difference between being a Vegetarian and being a vegan.

As mentioned earlier, veganism involves the complete expulsion of any kind of dairy/animal product from one's diet. However, vegetarianism allows some degree of freedom and flexibility to the diet and often allows animal-derived products such as milk and egg.

Keep in mind that this book has been designed to illustrate the VEGAN lifestyle specifically.

7 Reasons to go Vegan

"Why are you Vegan?" Anyone who has chosen to live on a vegan meal plan is very familiar with this question. It can even sometimes be an intimidating question as those asking it can often be rather antagonistic when asking. They also will often have their assumptions about why you choose to be Vegan and can be entirely wrong.

In 2002, a study showed that in the United States about 0.2% of Americans self-reported as being Vegan. That number has risen to close to 1% or even 1 1/2% as of late. Although still a very small number, that is an impressive upturn. What are the reasons for the increasing popularity of the Vegan diet? Why do people choose to be Vegan?

A couple of years back, I was the head of a Vegan support group that met on a monthly basis. Of our members, there were many different reasons why people were choosing the Vegan diet. Some people had several reasons overlapping, and some people had one, strong reason. In the media today, you can see these reasons popping up over and over. It seems to boil down to about seven main reasons that people are choosing the Vegan diet.

I find all of the reasons to be reasonable and fascinating. There seems to be something very freeing in following a diet and lifestyle based on conscientious choices. Perhaps it's the reality that when your mind is choosing what you eat rather than your appetite, it gives you a sense of control and power. It allows you to feel that you've taken the reins and are the master of your destiny. The following seven reasons seem to be primary in this conscious decision making:

1 Vegan Reason: Health

Although listed as number one in the list, it may or may not necessarily be the #1 reason people choose Veganism. I'm not aware of a study that has been done to determine this rank. However, health is one of the strongest reasons people are choosing the Vegan diet and is one of the most publicized reasons found today in the media and for a good reason. Over and over again, the Vegan diet has been proven to be one of the most healthful diets, if not THE most healthful.

2 Vegan Reason: Environmental Concerns

Today, more and more people are sharing a growing concern over the destruction of our environment. It is perhaps the greatest concern being discussed. Solutions to the problem are vast and varied, ranging from recycling to carpooling, to getting rid of the vehicles depending on unrenewable fuels. Interestingly, a Vegan diet ranks very high on ways to reduce your carbon footprint.

3 Vegan Reason: Animal Compassion

One of the most debated reasons for becoming Vegan is also one of the most strongly defended. The topic of animal cruelty is a hot one. Many Vegans may not have health concerns or environmental concerns, but they have a genuine heart for animals, and this reason alone is enough for them to make lifelong decisions to avoid any product relying on animals or animal byproducts. They not only adopt a Vegan diet, but also refuse to wear, purchase, endorse, or consume anything that in any way involves animal usage.

4 Vegan Reason: Religion and Spirituality

Just as there are many forms of Religion and Spirituality, there are many varied thoughts on what those Religions teach. Being most familiar with the Christian Religion, I find it interesting that some churches teach that it's Biblical to refrain from an animal-based diet and others teach that the Bible has declared all foods to be acceptable for our diets. It seems the same wide range exists in many other World Religions as well. In Buddhism, some sects lean toward Veganism, and some don't. One thing that seems consistent is that the question exists amongst most, if not all, of them.

5 Vegan Reason: Taste Preference

This reason is probably one of the most simple. It comes down to personal preference and, therefore, no-one is right or wrong. Some people like meat and dairy and some people don't. Although a simple reason, it is no less forceful to those who make Vegan choices based upon it.

6 Vegan Reason: Popularity and Uniqueness

More and more, the media is focusing on famous people who are making a turn to Veganism. The more this happens, the more people are following in their footsteps-especially young people. It is becoming more "hip" or non-traditional to break away from the standard "meat and potatoes" diet of the old days and to enter into the sleek and modern ways of Hollywood stars. For some, this reason alone is enough for them to make the change and stick to it.

7 Vegan Reason: Financial

In the United States, this single reason all by itself is probably not the reason people are changing to a Vegan diet, but it is a factor for many. In many third world countries, meat is a luxury. Often, the diet of these countries is more simple out of necessity and not out of choice. But, here in the United States, we tend to like to save a little money if we can. And those savings can be significant when choosing Vegan ingredients and recipes. This reason may be supplemental, but is a positive one.

The question "Why are you Vegan" is not as simple as it may seem. Vegans have many and varied reasons for their lifestyle. As we explore these reasons, I hope that you will gain more insight and awareness on the issues that prompt Vegan choices.

Different Types of Vegans

The different types of diets usually help people of different mindsets choose the one that best fits their preferred lifestyle. There are lots of different types of Vegan diet that all involve eating different things (while ALL involve NOT eating meat).

Some of the more prominent ones include:

- **Whole food Vegan Diet:** This is a diet that is based on a wide variety of different (whole) plant foods such as seeds, nuts, legumes, vegetables, fruits and whole grains.

- **Raw-Food Vegan Diet:** This diet is composed of raw fruits, nuts, vegetables, plant foods or seeds that are cooked under temperatures of 118 degrees Fahrenheit.

- **80/10/10:** This unique diet encourages an individual to rely on fat rich plants such as avocados and nuts and focuses more on raw fruits and tender greens. This diet is also known as "Fruitarian diet."

- **The Starch Solution:** This is similar to the aforementioned Fruitarian diet with the exception that it focuses on cooked starches such as rice, potatoes, and corn instead of raw fruits.

- **Raw Till 4:** This is a low-fat diet that is a variation of the fruitarian and Starch Solution diet. In this diet, Raw fruits are consumed up until 4 PM, after which, the individual has the option to cook a nice plant-based meal to end the day with.

- **Junk-Food Vegan Diet:** This diet relies largely on mock meats and vegan compliant cheese, desserts, and fries. Not to mention, other heavily processed vegan produces as well!

Despite the differences in such types of Vegan diets- the core objective remains the same.

"Get rid of meat, go for the greens!"

That will become the most important part of this book: Don't eat meat, and instead eat LOTS of greens. You should get most of your calories from vegetables, fruits, and nuts.

Vegan Food explained

There are thousands of different types of foods you could eat as a Vegan, such as:

- **Tofu, Seitan, and Tempeh:** These are excellent providers of proteins and are rich alternatives to fish, poultry, and meat.

- **Nuts and Nut Butters:** Go for pure unroasted and unblanched ones as they are packed with selenium, zinc, fiber, iron, etc.

- **Seeds:** Flaxseed, hemp, and chia are good choices when it comes to seeds as they are packed with a good dose of omega-3 fatty acids and protein.

- **Algae:** Chlorella and Spirulina are good choices when it comes to seeking out good sources of protein-packed Algae.

- **Calcium-Fortified Plant Milk and Yogurts:** These are excellent alternatives for a Vegan to meet their daily recommended calcium intake.

- **Nutritional Yeast:** Make sure to go for the ones that are labeled "Vitamin B12" as they are fortified for maximum benefit.

- **Sprouted and Fermented Plant Foods:** Produces such as tempeh, natto, miso, pickles, kombucha and Kimchi fall under this category, and they offer a good amount of vitamin K2 and probiotics.

- **Whole Grain Cereals and Pseudocereals:** These are good providers of complex carbs, iron, and Vitamin B.

- **Vegetables and Fruits:** These should make up the bulk of your diet. They are amazing sources of nutrients, and leafy greens including bok choy, kale, mustard greens and even spinaches are jam-packed with calcium and iron.

Food to avoid: This should be fairly self explanatory, but:

- Meat: Lamb, beef, horse, veal, organ meat, chicken, wild meat, goose, turkey, quail, duck, etc.

- Fish and Seafood: All types of seafood are restricted including squid, shrimp, anchovies, calamari, crab, etc.

- Eggs: Any eggs, including ostrich, quail, chicken, and fish are off the table.

- Dairy: Ice Cream, cheese, cream, milk, butter, etc. are restricted.

- Animal-Based Produce and Ingredients: For example whey, lactose, casein, egg white albumen, carmine, gelatin, etc. are to be avoided.

Now if this is your first time trying to go on a Vegan diet, the list mentioned above might discourage you to some extent. But don't let it! The advantages of being a Vegan more than makeup for the sacrifices that are made!

Benefits of consuming live plant-based foods

Here are some of the main benefits of going Vegan, just in case you've been scared off by the long list of things you can't eat that we just mentioned. Bare in mind that these are just a FEW of the many benefits of going Vegan, and many benefits you'll discover after just a few weeks:

- **Clear, supple skin:** Live plant-based foods are very rich in antioxidants, vitamins, and minerals which do a great job of eliminating toxic waste from your body and hydrating your skin; leaving you with beautiful and younger looking skin.

- **Sleep like an angel:** A plant-based diet is friendly to all your bodily functions. The same cannot be said of animal-based diets that usually overburden your digestive system meaning you don't get the required nutrition. The vegan diet ensures that your body functions optimally and when it comes to sleep time, you sleep like a baby as your bodily functions operate in the background.

- **Increased energy:** When your body is functioning optimally, thanks to a fresh and natural nutrient dense diet, you are sure to feel energetic with an increased mental focus.

- **Increased metabolic rate:** The vegan diet is exactly what man was meant to eat. As such, everything you eat that is vegan diet works to the benefit of your body including revving up your metabolism.

- **Decreased lethargy:** The vegan diet is the richest natural source of nutrients. This means that every part of your body is going to receive its required nutrition and so they will be no reason for you to feel deprived. The high fiber diet l keeps you full up to your next meal, and you don't need to worry about crazy hunger pangs, and the high amounts of water in the plant-based food keeps you hydrated all day.

The main thing is that you'll look better, feel better, and you'll be helping to save the planet and all the animals and humans on it.

What to actually eat on a vegan diet

Here are a few of the main things you should try and eat in your new Vegan diet, (don't worry, we'll explain more soon, and there will be recipes as well)

- **Fruits and veggies:** Apples, bananas, mangoes, berries, grapes, broccoli, leafy greens, carrots, variety of berries

- **Beans and legumes:** Lentils, lima beans, kidney beans, black beans, chickpeas, etc.

- **Whole grains:** Quinoa, rice, whole wheat, barley, rice, oats, etc.

- **Starch veggies and tubers:** Winter squash, potatoes, yams, celeriac, yucca, etc.

- **Nuts and seeds:** Almonds, cashews, walnuts, flax seeds, pumpkin seeds, hemp seeds, etc.

- **Superfoods:** Cacao, Spirulina, Goji Berries, Maca, Lucuma, Mesquite, Wheatgrass, Moringa

This is not an exhaustive list but the point to note is that the vegan diet is purely based on whole natural foods that have not been refined. A well-balanced diet will provide you with all the nutrition you need.

Avoid all animal-based foods and food products including cooking oil and also avoid refined food products that have very little nutrition. The goal here is to eat live plant-based foods that are bursting with healthy nutrition.

Getting enough protein and nutrients

There are a large number of people who will protest that Vegans don't get enough protein, or nutrients and things like Vitamin B12. This is a myth. Vegans get more than enough protein from vegetables and fruits, and Vitamin B12 can easily be supplemented.

- **Protein:** We don't eat fish, meat, poultry or other animal-based foods. These foods are high in protein which is important for our muscles and red blood cells. We need to find the best vegan substitutes that are also very high in protein such as:

- **Hemp Seeds:** At 35% plant-based protein with a full amino acid profile, this easily digestible and versatile seed is second to only…

- **Spirulina:** At 65%-75% protein by weight, this is the highest source of protein by weight compared to any other food.

- **Soy products:** Edamame, tofu and fortified soy drinks

- **Whole grains:** Buckwheat and quinoa

- **Legumes:** Beans, lentils and dried peas

- **Nuts and seeds:** Almonds, cashews, walnuts, flax seeds, sesame seeds, hemp seed, chia seeds

Getting enough Omega-3 fatty acids

These are essential for brain and heart health. It's important to eat these things. Let me repeat, to be healthy on a Vegan diet (and indeed, any diet) it's important to consume enough Omega

3 fatty acids, as these are what helps your brain function properly.

You can get them from:

- Natural oils: Flaxseed oil, canola oil, soybean oil, walnut and olive oil, hemp oil

- Ground walnuts and flaxseed

- Seeds: Hemp, chia seeds, flax, Sacha inch,

- Soybeans and tofu (*organic)

Omega 3 fatty acids are the things that when you get enough of them, you'll notice your brain firing on all cylinders. A great way to add them to your diet is to just have a few spoonfuls of ground flaxseed sprinkled on your cereal or mixed into your smoothie.

Getting the right Vitamins

Vitamins B12 and vitamin D help keep your blood cells and nerves healthy and also help your body absorb calcium. You can get these from:

- Fortified vegan meat alternatives

- Fortified drinks made from almonds, rice, and soy

- Red Star nutritional yeast

Minerals

Calcium, zinc, iron and other minerals are all very important for healthy and strong bones, a strong immunity and well-functioning body. You can get a healthy dose of minerals from:

Legumes, fresh fruits, sesame seeds, blackstrap molasses, fortified drinks, dried fruit such as prunes and whole grains.

Knowledge is key when getting into a vegan lifestyle. You need to know the right foods to eat and how to prepare great tasting meals.

How to start a Vegan diet, and change what you eat!

Many people around the world are making serious lifestyle changes to get their health back in good condition - and many of these people are doing this using the vegan diet. Yes, people are becoming increasingly aware of the amazing health benefits that this diet has to offer, but are often afraid of making the change.

How can they adopt veganism easily, without stress? The following tips are for those new to the vegan diet and are wishing to make a successful transition to the vegan lifestyle.

How to start a vegan diet:

Step 1 - Don't stress!

Stressing about the possible challenges and hardships of the vegan diet will not help you in any way, nor will it get you any closer to your goal. If you want to adopt the veganism lifestyle, (even if you are afraid a little) - DO NOT STRESS! This is an imperative tip for beginner vegans since many seem to stress too much and miss out of a lot of joy that this amazing journey has to offer!

Step 2 - You do not need to go vegan overnight.

Some folks can ditch their old lifestyle and adopt a new one overnight. I commend people like this, because this is something that many of us would like to do - but simply cannot. For the majority of folks, adopting a new lifestyle takes time, patience, and making small steps towards their goal. Do not despair if this is you!

Making a gradual transition to the vegan diet is advised.

As the famous saying goes, 'Slow and steady wins the race.' So making slow but constant changes to your diet will help slowly ingrain your new lifestyle into your brain, and you will be doing it at a comfortable, stress-free pace!

Giving yourself time to get used to the small steps and eliminations of the vegan diet is crucial for the beginner vegan!

The process of elimination

The following 7 foods should be eliminated, one at a time, at a comfortable pace: 1. Red meat. 2. White meat (chicken) 3. Fish & seafood. 4. Cheese. 5. Eggs. 6. Butter/cream. 7. Milk

If you slowly eliminate these foods, your transition to the vegan diet will be much more enjoyable and stress-free! As you reach each stage of elimination, you should endeavor to find some tasty recipes which accommodate your new dietary needs.

You can find many vegan/vegan transition recipes on the internet, either from websites, blogs, or professional vegan recipe e-books. For those new to the veganism lifestyle, finding tasty and easy-to-make recipes is a must to help keep you motivated and enjoying your food!

How to Stop Eating Dairy

It seems that stop eating dairy is one of the biggest challenges many people face when they start a vegan diet. Let's face it, there are so many products out there that contain dairy, and even in some products, the dairy is "hidden" from us by some by-products taken out from a dairy product.

I also struggled with this issue for a long time, and for me, it was more of a willpower issue than anything else. For periods of time, I would commit myself to stop eating any dairy products, and I would get the habit of reading labels to see that the product I was buying was 100% vegan.

But there were times in which my cravings for dairy products were very hard to handle. During these times I would say to myself that a little piece of cheese won't hurt, or an ice cream cone won't matter. Later I would find myself off track and with a great sense of guilt and try to commit myself to the vegan lifestyle once more. Repeating the cycle all over again.

So how can we stop that vicious circle of going on and off the vegan diet?

It comes down to retraining our desires and feelings as to what makes us feel good.

We might find comfort for a while in eating that ice cream cone, some cheese, or a piece of cake, but when you went vegan, you did it for a greater cause, and I hope you felt good once you made that choice.

It is no longer about what made you feel good in the past, but what makes you feel good now or in the long term. And to me, when I used to go back and forth between eating dairy, I noticed that I felt better not only physically but also emotionally when I went back to a vegan diet. That good emotion I felt every time I went back to a vegan diet grew stronger and stronger, helping me fight those cravings.

So now that you know what makes you feel good, you can consciously choose between that ice cream cone or that fruit. Once you make that conscious decision of choosing the fruit over the ice cream, you are breaking the cycle that pulls you out of your vegan. This in return will also make enormous improvements over your self-discipline as it will give you more power to choose the things that make you feel good.

Vegan muscle growth through nutrition

While most are happy with and look to achieve a trim belly and a healthy lifestyle, there are others who prefer to take things up a notch and tone their body by building muscle.

Before moving forward, let me clarify that there is a huge misconception that muscles cannot be adequately developed while on a Vegan diet! Vegans CAN and do build lots of lean muscle, and immense amounts of strength. It's not only possible, it's easy.

Aside from your regular muscle-building routine, there are certain key aspects of a vegan diet have in mind when ensuring that your muscles are developing and growing properly.

Building muscle as a Vegan (exercises, tips and tricks)

A lot of people have turned to Veganism either because it is healthy or because they feel bad about animals being killed. Some choose vegan diet as a way of life simply because it makes them feel better and energetic. Although vegan diet has limited choices when it comes to muscle building, there are a few diets and exercises that you can follow to acquire more muscles.

Oh, before we go any further, this section is optional for you, and if you DON'T want to build muscle, that's fine! Just don't do any of the exercises

I'm sharing in a second, or at least don't do them as much. Here comes the most important muscle building advice and tip of the century:

Whether you're on a Vegan diet or not, what you need to build muscle is a good combination of proteins, fat, and carbohydrates to build muscles along with a regular workout routine.

If you do not get this combination right, you will not be able to add any muscle, no matter how many green smoothies you drink in the morning.

The most important thing to remember is that you need to get enough calories in order to build muscle. Focus on counting your calories and making sure you're eating MORE than you need, through green smoothies, readybrek, vegetable soups and beans and rice.

Include surplus fresh vegetables and fruits along with fiber like oatmeal. Add healthy fats like olive oil, cheese to the daily diet. Fat is necessary for the recovery of muscles as well as maintaining the testosterone levels of the body which is necessary for muscle building so don't be scared to add it to your meals!

Although your diet menu is limited as a Vegan, you can compensate it by doing the more important part right. The most important part of any muscle building diet is to have the right food at the right time and not merely having the right food.

For example, if you have your proteins for the day immediately after your intense workout assuming that proteins are the ones that contribute to muscle building, you will be in for a shock! When done with your workouts, the muscle glycogen stored in the muscles would be depleted. Sugar has the property of secreting insulin, which acts as a catalyst to drive the consumed calories into muscle glycogen causing it to be stored as muscle. Hence, the ideal thing to have immediately after breakfast is a fruit juice or drink that is rich in carbohydrates sugar which leads to insulin secretion.

The next thing is your exercises. We've said that you need to eat enough calories, every day. The more you eat the more you'll grow. Now, for exercises, it really just needs to be kept simple:

Focus on constantly trying to lift heavier and heavier weights for SIZE.

Or focus on constantly building endurance and 'reps' for strength.

You can also mix these two for a combination of both. Generally, when you get bigger you also get stronger, but not always. So basically you just need to work out about 1-3 times a week, focusing on either exercises which target more than one muscle group (compound exercises) or exercises that focus on strength of one muscle group (like a dumbbell curl)

An example workout routine might look like this (for building size):

Monday:

- Some light cardio (a brisk walk or job, cycling etc)

- 3 sets of 6 reps of Benchpress at the max weight you can handle

- 3 sets of 6 reps of squats (with barbell, use a spotter, just below the ax weight you can handle)

Thursday:

- Some light cardio (swimming, cycling, Tai Chi)

- 3 sets of 6 pull-ups with a weight bag

- 3 sets of 6 reps of Deadlift (barbell, max weight you can handle AFTER cardio warmup)

And that's it! Keep eating the way you are (as a Vegan of course) and also, whenever you're doing something physical, give it ALL you've got. Go as hard as you can

because your body responds to that by growing stronger.

Essential Nutrients you need to know about

These are the nutrients which we consume to provide the energy required for our cells.

Protein: This is also known as the "building block of the body" since it helps to generate and heal different kinds of tissues in our body. It promotes growth and development.

Fat: While people often negatively look at fat, it is also essential as it acts as a backup reservoir of energy for the body.

Carbohydrates: Carbohydrates are the primary source of energy in our body.

Water: Water helps to maintain the optimum level of homeostasis in our body and is responsible for allowing the body to transport nutrients all around itself easily.

Minerals: Aside from the main nutrients, there are essential minerals that are needed in trace amounts to maintain a healthy body. For example, Potassium helps to maintain optimum cell fluid level, calcium strengthens the bones and so on.

Vitamins: Similar to minerals, vitamins are also needed in trace amounts to ensure that the body is functioning properly. Having a lack of certain vitamins often leads to a severe health problem. For example, Vitamin C is responsible for collagen synthesis, which helps to maintain the blood structure; on the other hand, Vitamin D helps to ensure that the body's calcium homeostasis level is maintained correctly.

The Basics of Protein

As you can already tell, protein is at the core of building your muscle. You will soon find out that meat is not the only source of good protein that is out there!

You must learn to appreciate the quality and effectiveness of protein. It is determined by a value that is called "Protein Digestibility-Corrected Amino Acid Score" (PDCAAS), which essentially compares the quality of protein amino acid with the requirements of a human and the ability of a human to digest it.

Eggs, for example, have a very high PDCAAS count, but since vegans are not allowed to eat eggs, it is essential that you know about different sources through which you will be able to get your protein.

Animal Vs. Plant Protein

There has been a long-standing debate between these two types of protein and their effectiveness when it comes to muscle building. Perhaps the core difference between animal and plant protein comes from the essential amino acids that are required by the body.

Animal proteins such as meat, eggs or dairy are similar to human beings' natural protein; thus, they are very easily absorbed. However, they are also high in LDL cholesterol and saturated fat, which might lead to harmful consequences in the long run.

Plant protein, on the other hand, is similar to animal protein, with the absence of just one or two essential amino acids for the body.

Regarding nutritional values, animal proteins tend to be very high in saturated fat and low in dietary fiber. Red meats have also been linked to some different health issues such as heart diseases and cancer. Alternatively, plant-based proteins tend to be lower in sodium and higher in fiber!

However, the problem when answering the question, "is vegan protein suitable for bodybuilding?" generally arises due to the difference between the amount of protein available in animal and plant protein.

For example, a cut of steak will provide you with approximately 40g of protein. Alternatively, a cup of tempeh will provide you with 31g of protein.

The answer to the question ultimately boils down to, "are you able to fulfill your daily protein intake (for bodybuilding) relying solely on vegetables?" The answer is yes. You might need to consume veggies in a more balanced and proper way, but it is indeed possible.

Is a Vegan Diet Safe?

The vegan diet has known for its amazing benefits and one of the best ways to prevent diseases in the long run. Many vegans have shared their experiences on this diet, and with an increasing number of vegan athletes and famous people joining the list, it is no doubt that this diet is going to remain a top choice for people wanting a better health and lifestyle.

But how safe is a vegan diet?

Along with many other diets, there are two sides of a coin. One side is the health benefits you can get by doing the vegan diet the right way, and the other is the unhealthy side of the vegan diet.

You need to understand that a change in your diet requires a lot more attention and knowledge on your part. You need to understand the type of nutrition your body needs and how to meet all those requirements in your new diet. Failure to do this can bring negative consequences.

If you think you can be a vegan and survive with just fruits and salads, then you are playing with fire.

Ensure that you pay close attention to your body and its nutritional needs in order to get maximum benefits. You need to become a student and learn more about nutrition. Get this right, and then you can start collecting all the benefits you get from a vegan diet.

To give you one advice right now, one of the major concerns you should have as a vegan is regarding vitamin B12. This vitamin is essential for the functioning of the brain and is a must for your health. Getting this vitamin requires proper planning, but it should not be hard to get. With so many fortified foods out there, you can find vitamin B12 in products such as soy milk, but remember it requires your attention.

So a vegan diet is safe if you know what you are doing. It may be tough but with practice and more knowledge, your vegan lifestyle is going to start getting easier and more enjoyable. Just don't give up on this diet and journey as the benefits are waiting for you.

The Dark Side of Veganism

Most people quickly identified a vegan diet with great benefits, not only regarding your health but also spiritual benefits such as compassion to all living things. So what is the dark side of veganism?

Some people find it very difficult and challenging to adopt a vegan lifestyle, and there are several reasons why they tend to fail. They have trouble finding accurate information, but even worse, they do not feel capable of making those changes in their diet.

Although it is possible to overcome this difficulty, people also tend to fail because they lack help from families, friends and they feel the environment takes a big toll on their failure too. They feel they cannot be vegan on a busy and fast pace life.

The biggest difficulty people have is giving up meat. This includes the most common such as beef, pork, chicken or turkey, but also meats such as fish, shrimp, ham, hot dogs and other similar foods. So for someone who always finds him or herself going to place to place without another choice other than a fast food meal, this can be quite challenging indeed.

Others find it very difficult to give up dairy. With products such as milk, cheese, yogurt and even ice cream on a hot summer day, people find it hard to give those up because it has been part of their diet since they were kids, so that brings another challenge as well.

And some people don't want to go as far as rejecting every product that may contain animal products such as leather, fur, silk. So if you are a person who loves fashion, this might also be a reason why adopting a vegan lifestyle is too hard.

It comes down to our domestication as a child to believe the certain myth about our diet that gets ingrained in our subconscious. For example, with all the research about all the hormones, pesticides and chemicals they put on our food, and consciously know about the health danger these products cause to our bodies, wouldn't be logical for everyone to become vegan?

If you want to adopt this diet, then one of the biggest things you need to have is willpower and commitment. Honor your word every day about your commitment to the vegan lifestyle and compassion to all living things. You might fall, but if you do, then commit yourself again to your veganism, and you will succeed.

Is Soy Bad for You?

There have been many controversies regarding the benefits of soy. Some scientists have shown the amazing benefits soy can bring to your health, while others claim that soy products contain toxins that are very harmful to our bodies.

People who claim that soy is bad for your health, are convinced that soy can bring side effects such as fertility problems for men, breast cancer, thyroid cancer and many other diseases.

But what the real truth about soy?

It is hard to know what the real truth regarding soy is. This is because there is so much money involved in this topic that research can be easily be manipulated by big industries covering information to the public for monetary issues.

So it comes down to making an educated guess. If we look back in time, soy has been using for thousands of years by the Chinese and they have no problems regarding male virility (they are the largest population on earth), and also China has the one of the lowest rate of breast cancer in women.

Now it is also important to buy soy products that are organic. With the high demand for soy in products, people have been discovering ways to make this product available at all times. Scientists have been manipulating with soy to make products that are just not healthy nor natural. Such is the case of isolated soy proteins, in which scientists put the soybean through so many processes that the result is completely synthetic. Products that contain isolated soy proteins can be found on energy bars, protein powders, and supplements hence look at the label so you could avoid it.

I support the idea that everything we consume, needs to be in moderation, (for example you can drown by drinking too much water) and always having a varied diet is a must.

If you think soy is bad for you, that should not stop you from becoming a vegan, as you can get your protein needs from many plant sources. For me, I like to keep soy on my diet as I do believe in its benefits but as I said before, everything must be done in moderation.

Vegan diet for better skin

The secret behind healthy skin is almost always your diet. You must follow healthy eating habits and stop eating junk basically. If you have been eating too much of oily and fried foods, stop them immediately. Your face can only look dull and drained with all these junk foods inside your body.

Water, green leafy vegetables, and salads, fish and skin hygiene, are the things you must eat lots of. A good and bright face should not be compromised, and you must follow a well-balanced diet and some tips to take care of your face. Here are some essentials for maintaining clear skin:

- **Water:** Water hydrates your dry and dull face. It is good to retain moisture in your face to make it glow all day long. It makes one look younger than their age. Age old secret behind a younger looking face is lots of water every day. 8-10 glasses of water are required for all body functioning too.

- **Food rich in antioxidants**: Any colorful vegetables such as carrot, beetroot are good. Spinach and carrot have antioxidants which are helpful to free radicals off your face. It also provides elasticity to your face and makes them supple.

- **Vitamin A, C, B and E:** Green leafy vegetables, carrot, beans and other fruits are rich in vitamins and minerals. Vitamin A, C, B, and E is very essential for overall growth of the cells and regeneration. Oranges especially have plenty of Vitamin C which prevents aging. You look young even at the age of 40 and 50. Eat plenty of salads and vegetables raw to retain the enzymes in them. Enzymes help digestion, and good gut health also reflects in your face. People who have suffered from constipation problems often see pimples and other eruptions. Keep your stomach clean!

By the way, you'll notice that just by switching to a Vegan diet, and stopping the consumption of dairy, eggs, and meat your skin will automatically become a lot clearer, sometimes even just within a week or so. That being said:

Try adding more water to your day by setting a reminder on your phone to drink every hour or so, and make sure that with your morning smoothies (recipes at the end of this ebook) add things like spinach, Vitamin C, and things like cucumber and Lettuce.

Vegan Diet and Disease control

A raw vegan diet can help control and massively reduce the risk of cancer, high blood pressure and the blood sugar level of diabetics, both type 1 and 2. It can even remove the need of insulin forever, or for as long as the raw diet goes on. This is not a miracle; it is only a natural way of living and eating, a simple cure which does not include harmful foods and does give the body what it needs so that it can process food and sugar normally.

The foods we eat literally construct and FORM our body.

It is normal that bodies which are given good food will be great constructions, as it is normal that bodies which are given bad foods (poor materials) make poor constructions. An example of a poor material to eat is sugar.

The nice thing about eating a raw vegan diet is that there is nothing harmful, in any quantities, in raw organic vegan foods. One can't develop cancer or asthma eating too many cucumbers or carrots, but one does develop both cancer and asthma eating too much dairy and meat products.

Removing the bad stuff is essential. There will be less need for insulin if there is no daily intake of triple chocolate cake and ice cream. Even though there are carbohydrates in a raw diet, it doesn't contain any poison fast sugars, and so the blood sugar level of a raw vegan food eater is necessarily easier to control than the blood sugar level of a normal North American eater.

A raw vegan diet includes precious enzymes which help rebuilt the pancreas of people with diabetes.

But this not all! A raw vegan diet doesn't only remove the bad stuff from our diet. It also adds something of critical importance to our body's health: Enzymes.

Enzymes are what keep us alive, the workers accomplishing pretty much everything: keeping the toxins out, building proteins, transporting precious nutrients in our blood, destroying cancers-to-be, boosting our immune system, helping us move, and probably think, feel, etc.

Every living thing is pretty much alive, thanks to enzymes. But every living thing has a limited amount of enzymes. No enzymes, no life. And so living things die when they have no more enzymes. Sounds crazy and even silly, but it's useful to know.

Animals have two types of enzymes: endogenous (coming from the body) and exogenous (coming from outside the body). Our body has two types of enzymes: digestive and metabolic.

Digestive enzymes digest foods, and metabolic enzymes do everything else.

When digestion is too hard, metabolic enzymes need to stop working on metabolic matters and come to help the poor overloaded digestive enzymes, leaving metabolic unresolved issues; this is the beginning of diseases. It is important to understand that enzymes contained in the food we eat help the work of our digestive enzymes, which need less help from metabolic enzymes.

Heat destroys almost 100% of all enzymes. We have the choice to eat living foods, full of them, or dead foods, harder to digest. Eating living foods will free the metabolic enzymes from digestive matters, and help them work on important health matters, hence helping the pancreas (which creates enzymes).

I know this might seem a bit confusing, but what I'm basically saying is that the more you COOK food, the more of the enzymes you destroy. By eating as much RAW food as you can, meaning vegetables, fruit etc, the more healthy enzymes you consume.

The more healthy enzymes you consume, the stronger your immune system will become, and the less likely it is that you'll get ill. It's that simple! Of course, sometimes you will have to cook food, and don't get me wrong, cooked vegetables and foods aren't BAD, they're just not AS GOOD as raw veggies and fruits.

The Amazing Benefits of Almond Milk

Almond milk is another proof to people who still don't want to leap a vegan diet either because they are allergic to soy, and wrongly believe that soy is the only protein choice for vegans, or because they don't like the taste of soy in milk or other products.

The benefits this milk can bring to your diet are amazing. Almond milk is a really good source of magnesium, manganese, selenium and some companies still enrich their almond milk with calcium, protein, and vitamins. Also, unlike cow's milk, almond milk contains a good amount of unsaturated fats, which helps in reducing the risk of heart disease.

What I have found great about almond milk it's the texture and flavor. The texture resembles a lot of that in cows milk, which is great if you want to do shakes, and the taste is very fresh and light. Also, I like to have almond milk in my fridge to add variety in my diet, which gives me a break from consuming soy milk.

One of the major concerns about almond milk at the beginning was the amount of sugar it has. Naturally, almond sugar does not contain any sugar, but to add taste to the milk, manufacturers started adding sugar, about 20 grams of sugar per serving, but luckily enough and with more demand for a more natural milk, you can now find almond milk with no sugar added. Ensure buying to make sure that the milk you are buying does not contain sugar.

So there you go, if you didn't like the taste of soy milk and that was stopping you from adapting to a vegan diet, try this type of milk. I have found it to be very useful in some recipes I have that include milk and what I like a lot of this milk is the vitamins and minerals it contains. Also, keep in mind that as the market grows. There is new alternative to milk such as rice milk, so keep an eye open for more vegan milk substitutes.

You should consume almond milk ideally every morning with a smoothie and use it to add liquid that you would normally have used dairy milk for.

Losing weight as a Vegan

Aside from eating fiber-rich veggies and fruits, the following tips will greatly increase the effectiveness of your diet!

When undergoing a vegan transformation, initially it will be really hard to resist the temptation of meat. Building up a very strong mental mindset that you are not allowed to eat meat is important. Embrace the absence of meat head-on. This will make your vegan journey easier.

Don't increase your intake of desserts and bread just because they are "Vegan compliant." Cut them down to one portion, and especially avoid sodas!

Try to go for high-protein and low-fat smoothies to keep your muscles pumped up- avoid fruit juices. They will help to gush the essential nutrients faster. Just make sure to replace the base milk with non-dairy products such as unsweetened soy milk.

Make sure to cut back on your sugar intake too; as it will make it much harder for you to lose weight.

If you plan to lose weight, then go for green leafy vegetables such as Bok Choy, Collard Greens, etc. They will provide you with a good dose of calcium, which will make your weight loss effort more efficient.

Keep in mind that simply eating veggies won't trim down your weight if you just sit around all day! Try to get some aerobic exercise to maximize your effort. Even a 30-minute treadmill walk will do! Just make sure to do a warm up session of 15 minutes before starting your exercise.

I'm a Vegan but I'm not losing weight?

If losing weight was your objective when choosing a vegan diet or if you are not a vegan, but losing weight is your main motivation to become one, then there are some myths we need to uncover so you won't feel cheated when trying out this diet and not seeing results.

You might have noticed that vegans do tend to be slimmer and it is very rare to see an overweight vegan, but sometimes that is not the case. Although vegans are hardly overweight, some people have trouble losing weight on a vegan diet.

Now we have heard the formula before, the one that tells you that to lose weight you need to burn more calories than what you take, which I truly believe is true and it really makes sense, but there are cases in which people eat way less than another individual, yet they gain weight, and the other person doesn't. We need to understand that people have different bodies and metabolisms, and some have bodies that can burn fat faster than others. If you have this type of metabolism, then you need to pay close attention how many calories you get.

Physical activity is an extremely important factor if you want to lose weight. If you live a life in which you drive to work, work in an office, spend some time in front of the TV at night, there are great chances that your unwanted weight comes from your physical inactivity.

So it is important to exercise at least for 15 mins a day. If you feel like you don't have time, start organizing your agenda to make space for that 15 min of exercise, and along with the vegan diet, you will start to see amazing results.

Now if you want to see results even faster, I will recommend you see a nutritionist so they could give you a diet, vegan of course, along with some tips on exercise and they will help you keep track of the progress you are making and push you to attain greater results.

If you keep up with the vegan diet, I can guarantee you that you will reach your desired weight if you are persistent enough. By following a vegan diet, one of the really good benefits you will get is your higher fiber intake. Current recommendations for fiber intake are 27-40 grams. Vegans meet and even exceed this recommendations by taking an average of 40-50 grams. This benefits you in your quest for better weight because fiber helps in your digestive system, better bowel movement, reduces hunger and improves satiety.

Use Veggies, Fruits, and Exercise for Weight Loss and See How It Helps

The subject of weight loss or plan to enter into this phenomena is a very tedious and cumbersome exercise. If you are determined and motivated to healthily cut down your fat especially around your waistline or belly, then there is no looking back to make your body slim, smart and full of liveliness.

Excess weight is the leading causes of death in the world as it leads to many diseases such as:

1. Diabetes.

2. Heart Disease.

3. Hypertension.

4. Liver Disease.

5. Sleep Apnea.

6. Osteoarthritis.

The easiest, the first and foremost way for weight loss is to drink plenty of water and make sure you get habitual about drinking water and exercising.

We have water abundantly around us. It is water that flushes our bodies, and of course, it has zero calories. The first thing to do in the morning after brushing your teeth is to take a glass full of lukewarm water, also try to drink it with every meal. Avoid coke, and other soda drinks as these have very high calories and for sure disturb your metabolism.

Eating habits help in fat reduction and vice versa. Do not skip your meal especially breakfast, if you skip your breakfast you are bound to eat more at lunchtime thus adversely affecting your weight loss campaign.

Fresh fruits and vegetables is a perfect solution for your weight loss plan, so pick those which have comparatively low sugar contents such as tomatoes, lettuce, broccoli, carrot, papaya, orange, apple, and watermelon, all these vegetables have low calories but are high in protein, as these are natures produce so take maximum benefit of out of this.

Workouts and weight loss go together, so do not drag your feet on this, and start your exercises now. But you should choose what and which exercise will suit your age group, hence consult your doctor. Jogging and long-running is the best exercise and most effective ways to burn your calories and tremendously helps in weight loss.

If you cannot jog or run go for a brisk walk, it will keep you fit and agile. Aerobic training in a small group is very helpful; breathing exercises are the best, you can do these exercises at any time and anywhere and as such no special gear is required for this job.

Deep fried foods for obese people are fully restricted as these contain very high measure cholesterol and carbohydrates, both of these are harmful to overweight people and are bound to compound the problem.

One more product that helps in this matter are herbal teas, but it should be used regularly, the process of burning fat with this product may consume some time, but it has no side effects and is very valuable.

Smoothie recipes for a faster brain and a better body

Now, before we start this section, bare in mind that some of the best ways to get calories, is to drink them. Drinking calories in the form of smoothies makes it easier to get your calories up (which is good for building muscle) and also get your vitamins and nutrients in, easily.

The best part about smoothies, is that they're quick, easy, and you can just add whatever you want to eat to them. If you need to get more Omega 3s, just add some more flaxseeds to your smoothie. Need more protein? Add more almond milk or spinach.

The best way to approach this section is to just try a different smoothie every few days. Make the ones that appeal to you most, and remember, you can always add things to taste, for example bananas and spinach are great ingredients to add to make it smoother and more sweet tasting.

Here are some power smoothie recipes that can help you boost your brainpower and feel better and stronger:

1. Chocolate Green Smoothie

Preparation time: 5-10 minutes

Ingredients

1/2 cup of sliced apples of choice

3/4 cup coconut cream

100g spinach chopped

1/4 cup cocoa powder

3-4 Squares of 85% dark chocolate

2-3 drops of stevia sweetener

Directions

1. Put everything in a blender and blend till smooth!

2. Enjoy!

2. Choco-Berry Cheesecake Smoothie

Preparation time: 5-10 minutes

Ingredients (per serving)

¼ cup cashew cheese

¼ cup coconut milk

½ cup frozen raspberries

1 tbsp. cacao powder

¾ cup water

1 tbsp. Extra virgin coconut oil

4 drops liquid Stevia extract

Directions

1. Blend the ingredients and pulse away

3. Chocolate Berry Avocado Smoothie

Ingredients

1 1/3 cup Cashew Milk

1/2 avocado

1/3 cup frozen raspberries & blueberries

1 tbsp cocoa powder

3 drops of stevia

1/8 tsp blueberry extract

Directions

1. Blend the ingredients and pulse away

4. Blackberry & Raspberry Vegan Cheesecake Smoothie

Preparation time: 5 minutes

Ingredients (per serving)

½ cup blackberries & Raspberry

¼ cup full-fat coconut milk

¼ cup heavy whipping coconut cream

½ cup water

1 tbsp MCT oil

A few drops of Vanilla

4 drops liquid Stevia Extract

Directions

1. Add ingredients to blender and pulse.

5. Spring Redcurrant Smoothie

Preparation time: 5 minutes

Ingredients (per serving)

½ cup redcurrants, fresh or frozen

2 large Fresh strawberries

¼ cup coconut milk

½ cup water

3 tbsp. chia seeds

½ vanilla bean

4 drops liquid Stevia extract

Directions

1. Blend the ingredients and pulse away until smooth Also please allow to set and settle a little bit!

6. Fresh Keto Berry Shake

Preparation time: 5-10 minutes

Ingredients

¼ cup creamed coconut milk

½ cup almond milk

½ cup fresh mixed berries

1 tbsp. MCT oil

½ cup ice

4 drops Stevia extract

½ tsp vanilla extract

Whipped Coconut Cream on top

Directions

1. To cream, the coconut milk just allows coconut milk can in the refrigerator overnight the spoon it a hard solid piece of coconut milk and

throw away liquids. Make sure not shake before opening.

2. Add ingredients in a blender and pulse.

3. Serve when smooth after a pulse.

7. Coconut Vegan Strawberry Smoothie

Preparation time: 5-10 minutes

Ingredients

¾ cup strawberries Fresh or Frozen

1 cup of coconut milk

2 tablespoons smooth cashew butter

2 packets stevia or 3-4 drops stevia drops

Directions

1. Add all ingredients in a blender.

2. Then Blend!

3. And Enjoy!

8. Low-Carb Strawberry & Rhubarb Pie Smoothie

Preparation time: 5 minutes

Ingredients

2 medium strawberries

1 medium rhubarb stalks

2 tbsp. almond butter

2 tbsp. of chia seeds

½ cup almond milk

3 tbsp. coconut milk

1 tsp thinly grated fresh ginger root

½ tsp pure vanilla bean extract

5 drops liquid Stevia extract

Directions

1. Blend the ingredients and pulse away

2. Enjoy!

9. Keto Frozen Mint Hot Chocolate

Ingredients

1 cup unsweetened almond milk

3-4 ounces dark chocolate 90%, chopped

1/2 cup Brown Rice Protein powder

1/2 tsp peppermint extract

1 tsp liquid stevia

1½ cups ice

Directions

1. Add all ingredients in blender and pulse.

2. Optional: Top With Whipped Coconut Cream!

10. Chocolate Macadamia Smoothie

Preparation time: 5-10 min

Ingredients

1 1/3 cup ice cubes

2/3 cup coconut milk

3 tbsp. crushed macadamia nuts

3-4 Stevia drops

1 tbsp. unsweetened cocoa powder

1/2 tsp vanilla extract

Directions

1. Blend the ingredients into smooth.

2. Optional: Top with whipped coconut cream, and add crushed macadamia nuts.

11. Chocolate Almond Butter Milkshake

Preparation time: 5 min

Ingredients

¾ cup coconut milk

¾ tablespoon unsweetened cocoa powder

2 tablespoons Almond Butter

4 drops Stevia Drops

Dash Pink Salt

Directions

1. Place all ingredients in blender and pulse.

2. Enjoy!

12. Keto Cherry Chocolate Post Workout Smoothie

Ingredients

1/2 cup fresh pitted cherries

¾ cup coconut milk

1 scoop soy protein

½ cup hemp hearts

1/5 cup unsweetened cocoa powder

4 drops stevia drops

1 cup ice

2-4 pieces of 85% dark chocolate

Directions

1. Place all ingredients in blender and pulse!

2. Enjoy!

Chapter 18: Vegan Recipes for a faster brain

1. Mustard-Citrus Vinaigrette

Prep Time: 6 minutes

Yield: 6 tablespoons

Ingredients

2 tablespoons lemon juice

4 tablespoons olive oil

1/4 teaspoon sea salt

1/2 teaspoon Dijon mustard

Directions

1. In a bowl add the lemon juice.

2. Add the Dijon mustard, and olive oil.

3. Mix well and season with sea salt.

2. Almond Keto Mousse

Ingredients

13.5 oz coconut milk

1/4 tsp. liquid stevia

2 Tbsp. almond butter

Directions

1. Add the coconut milk into a bowl.

2. Add the almond butter and liquid stevia.

3. Whisk well to make a smooth mix.

4. Add to desired cups and freeze for 1 hour.

3. Raw Herb Inspired Veggie "Pasta"

Serves: 5

Prep time: 8 minute

Ingredients

4 Tbsp. Antioxidant Omega Oil Blend

1 tsp dried oregano

2 cloves garlic, diced

2 zucchini, peeled, cut into strands

2 tsp fresh rosemary

1 Tbsp. shredded fresh basil

2 tsp dried basil

Salt and pepper, to taste

Directions

1. In a mixing bowl combine the garlic, rosemary, basil, and oregano.

2. Mix well and season using salt and pepper.

3. Add the oil blend and mix well.

4. Finally, add the zucchini strands and toss gently.

5.   Serve fresh.

4. Cashew Cheese Veggie Bites

Makes 14-16 Servings

Ingredients

1 cup almonds

3 tablespoon fresh lemon juice

1 cucumber, cut into thick slices

1 clove garlic, minced

Pinch of salt

1 teaspoon yeast

1 tomato, diced

1/4 cup cashews

Cayenne Pepper

Directions

1. Soak the nuts in water for about 4 hours and then make a paste out of them.

2. Add the cayenne pepper, salt, yeast, garlic and lemon juice with the nut pastes.

3. Mix well.

4. Arrange the cucumber slices on a tray and add the nut paste, tomato and serve.

5. Roasted Mushroom Mix

Ingredients

1 teaspoon of balsamic vinegar

2 pounds of mixed fresh mushrooms

1/2 cup of olive oil

2 garlic cloves, minced

1 teaspoon of minced fresh sage

Salt and pepper to taste

1/4 cup of minced fresh parsley

1 teaspoon of minced fresh rosemary

Directions

1. Rub the mushrooms with a cleansed and moist cloth. Preheat the oven to 350 degrees F.

2. Clip the stems of the mushrooms.

3. Dice them into 2" pieces. In a large ovenproof casserole, combine olive oil with the garlic, fresh herbs and favoring ingredients. Roll in the mushrooms and mix well.

4. They should be covered with the seasoned oil. Bake for 30-40 minutes. Take out from the oven and drizzle the balsamic vinegar. Serve.

6. "Pasta" Alfredo

Ingredients

For the pasta

2 zucchinis (shaped in spirals)

For the sauce

1 cup of almond milk

1 T of lemon juice

1 head of a cauliflower

3 T of nutritional yeast

3 cloves of garlic, chopped

Salt to taste

2 T of onions diced

Directions

1. Slit the cauliflower into florets and boil till they become tender.

2. With the help of a peeler, mandolin or spiralizer dice the zucchinis into strips.

3. Now using a food processor or blender, mix up the boiled florets and other ingredients.

4. Top the zucchini pasta with this sauce and dish out instantly.

5. If you plan to dish out later then keep the zucchini pasta and sauce in two different bowls.

7. **Nutty & Spicy Dip**

Prep Time: 5 minutes

Cooking Time: 5 minutes

Ingredients

1 cup of almond milk

1/2 teaspoon of chili powder

1/4 teaspoon of smoked paprika

1 cup of raw almonds

1/2 cup of nutritional yeast

1/4 teaspoon of garlic powder

Pepper and cayenne to taste

1/4-1/2 teaspoon of sea salt

Directions

1. Mix up all the ingredients in a high-speed blender or food processor.

2. Preserve in the freezer topped with a lid in a suitable food container.

3. You can mix up any spice or a variety of flavors as per your choice.

8. Cinnamon Maple Almond Butter

Ingredients

1 tablespoon of pure maple syrup

3/4 cup of natural almond butter

1/4 teaspoon of ground cinnamon

3/4 cup of vanilla almond milk

Directions

1. In a blender or food processor, mix up all the ingredients smoothly.

2. Save in the freezer in a bolted container.

3. Yields 1 and 3/4 cups.

Conclusion

Changing your diet, especially one that it been proven to give you so many health benefits in the long and short-term can be an exciting and fun time in your life. You're on an incredible journey, and by following the tips and ideas in this book, you'll be able to supercharge your body.

I'd advise to start trying the recipes found towards the end of this guide, maybe try a new one every few days and see what you feel like afterwards. The best way of working out what's the best thing to eat is to really listen to your body.

For example, with the smoothies, just try one in the morning and notice how you feel throughout the day. I find that the best smoothies are the ones that taste great, and give me energy not just for the first hour but for the first 5 hours of the day.

Remember that it this is also the time in which you need to put a little more effort and time in knowing what decisions to make to follow the right path. You need to trust yourself, and just believe that this is the best thing to do for you, your health, and the health of the word.

Most people who decide to go vegan will have a lot of success for the most part. They understand that working to be healthy is not impossible, but it will require time to know this diet inside and out. When adopting a vegan diet, you need to become aware of the nutrients you need and how to replace those nutrients, the ones you got from animal products, with a plant-based diet. It is essential to know foods you are eating and also what you are missing, as this is critical to your success as a vegan.

At the beginning is also better to consult with your doctor or nutritionist, as they will help you to identify what nutrients your body needs the most and will guide you through a vegan diet that fits your needs.

This is important because you might not know which nutrients you are lacking, or which ones are the most important to you and your needs until your doctor determines the type of condition you are currently in.

Lacking knowledge of proper nutrition might complicate your journey as a vegan, which done properly, shouldn't hard. So always seek to achieve proper nutrition in your vegan diet as this will help you not only achieve better health, but also optimal energy levels throughout the day.

So a bit of effort at the beginning could yield you years of good health and balance in your life. Just take the time to know your needs better and try to cover them with a plant-based diet. Nowadays it's easy to find products from all over the world, so it's not impossible to live on a plant-based diet.

Do this, and your journey as a vegan would be the best choice you have made towards your health.

Thanks for reading, now go and save the world!

Disclaimer:

A word should be said on nutrition and advice. Please note that by reading this book, you agree and accept that this does not constitute nutritional or health advice, and that you take full resonsibility for any foods or drinks that you do or do not consume. This is intended to be for educational purposes only, and not for licensed medical advice.

Always consult with your GP or physician before making any lifestyle or dietary changes, and always do your own independent research before changing your diet in any way.

Copyright:

This book was produced by **TranscendYourLimits.com** and should not be resold anywhere except the website and other agreed outlets. You do not have permission to copy, redistribute or otherwise modify any of the contents in this book.